Pau d'Arco

(Taheebo, Lapacho)

Rita Elkins, M.H.

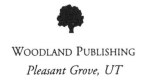

Woodland Publishing
Pleasant Grove, UT

Woodland Publishing
P.O. Box 160
Pleasant Grove, UT
84062

CONTENTS

PAU D'ARCO

INTRODUCTION

Pau d'arco, also commonly known as *taheebo* and *lapacho,* has a fascinating history and is considered one of the world's most unique therapeutic botanicals. While it is referred to as an herb, its classification as a tree bark technically relegates it to another category. Relatively new to Western herbalists, pau d'arco is harvested from the inner bark of the hardy lapacho tree, which is native to South American regions of the Andes mountains. The lapacho tree is famous for its extremely hard wood and unusually deep roots. The red lapacho tree bears brilliant scarlet flowers and also thrives in the tropical lowlands, resisting fungal growth.

The name *taheebo* refers to the inner bark of the lapacho tree, which has become quite famous for its extraordinary medicinal uses. In the last few decades, its ability to treat systemic yeast infections has brought it to the attention of American herbalists. Reports of dramatic cancer cures in South America have also engendered an enormous amount of interest in pau d'arco. As clinical data begins to mount, the use of pau d'arco tea for numerous health problems is becoming more common in this country. Harvested in the Andes regions of Brazil and Argentina, pau d'arco, like other tropical forest plants, has a long history of medicinal applications and is one of many marvelous botanicals whose therapeutic uses has remained relatively untapped.

PAU D'ARCO

(*Tabebuia avellanedae*)

FAMILY: Bignoniaceae (*Note:* Dozens of different species of the family Bignoniaceae exist. Over 100 *Tabebuia* species are native to tropical America alone. They are usually identified by their leaf configuration and flower color. Trees that bear red, violet or pink flowers are usually preferred for their medicinal value. The name *ipes* applies to many species of the genera *Tabebuia*. There are at least four species that are considered true lapacho and include: *Tecoma orchracea, T. Ipe, Tabebuia cassinoides* and *T. avellandedae.*)

Herbalist Terry Willard states that "the taxonomy of this genus is very difficult. It is quite possible that there is confusion among even trained gatherers. One specific way of distinguishing the species is at the seedling stage. The 4-leave clover-like cotyledons are distinctly deeply cleft. Some have taken seed from a stand, grown seedlings to assure the species of the stand, assuring the highest medicinal quality."[1]

The *Tabebuia avellandedae* is considered one of the largest trees in the forests near Sao Paolo, Brazil, and is considered the true "lapacho." It takes more than twenty years for these trees to mature. A search for pau d'arco or taheebo sources has found that Argentina and Brazil grow more of these trees than any other South American countries.

COMMON NAMES: pau d'arco, palo de arco, taheebo, ipes, ipe roxo, lapacho, *T. ipe, T. cassinoides, Tecoma curialis, Tecoma orchracea,* trumpet bush, divine tree

Pau d'Arco

PLANT PARTS: inner bark of lapacho tree

HARVESTING METHODS: Pau d'arco is harvested by peeling the bark of the lapacho tree in vertical strips from the ground up to approximately six feet. Only the inner bark is pharmacologically active. The process of separating the inner from the outer bark can be slow and painstaking. The bark strips are subsequently cut into pieces and dried.

CHEMICAL CONSTITUENTS: volatile oils (trace); phenols and phenolic glycosides; tannins; pseudo-tannins (chrysophanic acid); quinones (naphthoquinones, anthraquinones); saponins; steroid saponins (beta sitosterol)

ACTIVE COMPOUNDS: Pau d'arco is considered a bitter herb with sixteen quinones (naphthoquinones, anthraquinones) including tabeuin, a newly discovered compound. The napthoquinones exert a highly effective action against certain infections, especially those of the *Candida albicans* variety. Pau d'arco extracts also contain benzoic acids and quercitin. Lapachol comprises the major chemical constituent of pau d'arco. In most cases, the quality of the pau d'arco is based on its content of lapachol. The following was reported in *Cancer Chemotherapy Reports:*

> Quinones play significant roles in many areas of chemistry and biochemistry and many derivatives have been synthesized for study. Because of their availability and the biologic properties known to be associated with the quinone structure, a large number of these compounds have been screened over the past 17 years in the NCI's [National Cancer Institute] Drug Research and Development program aimed at the discovery of leads to new classes of antitumor drugs.[2]

Anthraquinones include:

- 2-methyl anthraquinone
- 2-hydorxy methy lanthraquinone
- 2-acetoxy methyl anthraquinone
- anthraquinone-2-aldehyde
- 1methoxy anthraquinone
- 1-hydroxy anthraquinone
- 2-hydroxy-3-methyl quinone
- tabebuin

Napthoquinones include:

- lapachol
- menaquionone-1
- deoxylapachol
- alpha-lapachone
- beta-lapachone
- dehydro-alpha-lapachone

Studies conducted in 1974 stated in *Cancer Chemotherapy Reports* that "lapachol has been shown to have antimalarial activity in animals and is a known uncoupler of oxidative phosphorylation. More recently, [lapachol] was found to have antitumor activity . . ."[3]

PHARMACOLOGY: The particular blend of quinones found in pau d'arco is quite rare. It is lapachol, a naphthoquinone which is considered vital to the antimicrobial action of pau d'arco.

Lapachol is considered the first active compound of pau d'arco to be clinically studied. Extracts of the bark have shown antitumor activity.[4] Quercitin, a bioflavonoid and benzoic acids are also contained in the heartwood of the tree.[5] Pau d'arco contains high amounts of iron and calcium, as well as selenium vitamin C, vitamin A, B-complex vitamins, potassium, sodium, and zinc.

Pau d'Arco

CHARACTER: analgesic, alterative, antibiotic, anti-inflammatory, anti-malarial, antineoplastic, antioxidant, antiviral, antiparasitic, antipyretic (fever), antitumor, astringent, diuretic, laxative, tonic

ACTIONS: Pau d'arco is considered a potent disease-fighting botanical which supports the immune system.

HERBAL FORMS: Pau d'arco is usually administered in a decoction or tea which is consumed several times throughout the day. The bark should be boiled in a cup of water for 10 to 20 minutes or commercially prepared tea bags can be used. It is also available in an aqueous or solid extract. Topical applications in the form of ointments of pau d'arco have been used to treat vaginal yeast infections and skin diseases. *Using the whole plant is preferable to using only isolated compounds or ingredients.*

Like so many other therapeutic herbs and natural nutrients, tests have shown that attempting to isolate certain quinones like lapachol has not been as effective as using the herb in its entirety.[6] As is always the case with medicinal botanicals, using them in the form Mother Nature created is preferable. Synergistic effects which cannot be duplicated with isolated synthetic analogs are inherent to the pharmacology of any therapeutic herb.

SAFETY: Using pau d'arco in its whole plant form is not considered unsafe for human consumption. The FDA approved lapacho [pau d'arco] as safe for human consumption in 1981. The isolated lapachol component of pau d'arco has shown an anti-vitamin K activity, although due to its content of vitamin K-like compounds, this is not thought to be a problem. Continued therapeutic use of lapachol alone in laboratory animals produced varying degrees of anemia and other toxicity.[7] Concerning this toxicity, subsequent studies published in 1970 by Chas Pfizer & Co. found that all signs of lapachol toxicity in animals could be completely reversed.[8]

Using pau d'arco tea in its whole form rather than isolated lapachol compounds has been considered completely safe. No reports of toxicity in humans exist when decoctions of the bark are used.[9] Possible side effects which are not considered common include: laxative effect and mild nausea. Any side effects associated with taking pau d'arco have also been linked to cellular detoxification, which is not unusual when taking herbal preparations. Once the cells have been altered, side effects should diminish.

HISTORY

Pau d'arco is native to South American regions. Its bark is harvested from the lapacho tree, which grows up to 125 feet tall in the Andes Region of the country.[10] Most lapacho trees are found in Brazil, Argentina and Paraguay and are considered ozoniferous trees or trees which primarily grow in high ozone regions. Typically, air that has high ozone counts is fresh and free from pollution, exhaust, smoke, pesticides and other toxins.

The herbal component of this tree is found in its inner bark and is known by a variety of names. The origin of its name, which means "bow stick," comes from the practice of using the limbs of the lapacho tree to make archery bows. In Argentina, the herb is called "lapacho," in Brazil "ipe" and here in the United States it is most commonly known as "pau d'arco" or "taheebo."

For over a millennia, Brazilian Indians such as the Callaway tribe (descendants of Inca medicine men), have used the inner bark of the lapacho tree as a traditional folk remedy for various disorders and were the ones to originally name it *taheebo,* meaning "inner bark." According to local legends, these Indians discovered the healing properties of pau d'arco by following the example of animals indigenous to the region. Modern scientists have been intrigued by tribal medicinal practices and refer to their use of botanicals as the "Callaway Pharmacopoeia." Research has discovered that these Indians used (and continue to use) lapacho bark for arthritis, bed wetting, boils, colitis, constipation, cystitis, dysentery, fever, lung infections, prostate disorders, sore throats, snake bites and ulcers.[11] Both the tea and paste form of the bark have been used by Brazilian Indians for malignancies, especially skin cancer. The Guarani, Tupi and several other tribes call the lapacho tree "tajy," which means "to have strength and vigor" or "divine tree."[12] Because of its extraordinary medicinal powers it was subsequently referred to as the "treasure of the Incas."

Legends relate that the Vikings sold pau d'arco for its miraculous herbal powers and believed that it originated on the moon. The Czars of Russia reportedly drank pau d'arco tea for longevity, and Gandhi supposedly was a staunch believer in the therapeutic value of a daily cup.

South American Indians shared the healing properties of pau d'arco with early Portuguese and Spanish settlers who used it to treat a disease referred to as schistosomiasis. This particular disease was caused by a flatworm (trematode) which normally penetrated the body. Using pau d'arco prevented the parasite from entering the body. This antiparasitic effect was first observed with cut down lapacho trees that deteriorated in humid, tropical climates but did not become moldy or mildewed.

Lapachol, the active compound found in pau d'arco was first isolated in 1884 by E. Paterno. In 1896, S.C. Hooker arrived at its chemical configurations and in 1927, L.F. Fieser was able to synthesize the substance.[13] Even in the late nineteenth century, the healing powers of lapacho (pau d'arco) were recorded by several European physicians. These doctors were the first to approach the fact that the medicinal claims made concerning pau d'arco were based in science. Theodore Meyer of the national University of Tucuman in Argentina was the first modern scientist to study the chemical constituents of pau d'arco. Under his direction, pau d'arco or pau d'arco was distributed to cancer patients throughout Argentina. For over 10 years, Dr. Meyer tried to bring pau d'arco as a credible cancer treatment to the attention of the medical and scientific establishment. He amassed a great deal of impressive data supporting his view, however, because his methods were rather crude, much of his findings were dismissed. Dr. Meyer died in

1972 before his dream of establishing lapacho (pau d'arco) as a legitimate therapeutic agent occurred. However, interest in pau d'arco continued.

Research teams at the Universidade do Recife in Brazil discovered that the bark contained xyloidone, a compound with antiviral properties. Lapachol, another compound with anti-tumor activity was also isolated and studied in 1956 by researchers in Brazil. Since then, a quinone called tabebuin has also been discovered. Pau d'arco has been scientifically investigated over the last few decades. South American reports have been the most impressive. In 1967, scientists at the University of Aberdeen discovered 16 quinones, along with two benzoic acids and quercitin, a bioflavonoid.[14]

Dr. Orlando dei Santi began to prescribe pau d'arco to his cancer patients in Brazil after his brother was miraculously cured of cancer after taking lapacho [pau d'arco] therapy in 1960. Several other physicians became interested in pau d'arco and it was subsequently used to treat a number of cancer patients at the Municipal Hospital of Santo Andre in Brazil. In time, many dramatic stories of various cancer cures emerged and were published in local periodicals. Interestingly, as these reports circulated, the national government ordered all physicians to stop making any public comments about the curative properties of pau d'arco. It was Dr. Alec De Montmorency who finally came forward and published a complete report of Brazilian clinical trials conducted on pau d'arco. His review generated a great deal of worldwide curiosity and new interest in the herb.

Prats Ruiz, a general practitioner in the city of Concepcion, has also studied the use of pau d'arco for leukemia. He successful treated several cases of leukemia with pau d'arco in his private clinic. Dr. Paulo Martin, a researcher for the Brazilian government subsequently supported the notion that pau d'arco could also kill infections, even if they were viral. He stated, "We isolated a compound we called quechua from pau d'arco and found it to be a powerful antibiotic with virus-killing properties."[15] Dr. James Duke of the National Institutes of Health and Dr. Norman Farnsworth of the

University of Illinois confirmed Martin's claims, stating that pau d'arco contains a substance found to be effective against certain cancers.

According to Brazilian and American press reports, pau d'arco teas have been used to successfully treat a number of serious illnesses. The Santo Andre Hospital in Rio de Janeiro has used pau d'arco to treat cancer and other infectious diseases since the early 1970s. Various reports both anecdotal and otherwise support the notion that pau d'arco preparations have had some dramatic results in certain cancer patients, one being the brother of Dr. Orlando dei Santi, mentioned earlier. Subsequent tests at this hospital also suggested that pau d'arco may be of value for diabetics as well. As results emerged, several articles on the curative properties of pau d'arco were published in *O Cruzeiro*, a Brazilian magazine. Today, pau d'arco is sold as an over-the-counter herbal preparation and in pharmacies.

Clinical studies conducted in the 1970s and 1980s found that the lapachol component of pau d'arco had the ability to fight viral infections, parasites and a variety of cancers including leukemia. Because clinical data on the therapeutic benefits of pau d'arco has been accumulated in South American countries, U.S. research has begun but is still limited.

In 1968, extracts from pau d'arco were in phase 1 of pre-clinical screening by the National Cancer Institute in Bethesda, Maryland. Initial results suggested that the lapachol quinone of pau d'arco had promising anti-cancer properties due to its action against 256 Walker tumors.[16] In 1970, testing of lapachol as a new drug was suspended due to the fact that some deleterious side effects had been reported.[17]

Some health practitioners believe that isolating just the lapachol constituent of pau d'arco intensified any negative side effects, thereby implying that using the herb in its whole form was preferable and much more safe. Unfortunately, the National Cancer Institute did not investigate the whole plant, a policy which has caused several potentially life saving herbs to slip through the system.

Today, herbalists and other health practitioners use pau d'arco to treat herpes infections, diabetes, arthritis pain, cancer and hypoglycemia. Argentinean doctors continue to use pau d'arco and its extracts. It is one of several tropical forest botanicals which have been enthusiastically received in North America, Europe and Asia and may eventually emerge as a viable cancer treatment in this country. Pau d'arco's reputation has crossed international boundaries primarily through word of mouth. Recently, articles concerning its curative potential have been published in Sweden, Germany and Japan. As of yet, no official medical opinion concerning its therapeutic use has been issued in this country. Because of the AIDS epidemic, new interest in pau d'arco has recently emerged due to its documented antiviral properties.

OVERVIEW

While pau d'arco is very well known in South American countries, its curative powers have remained relatively unknown in this country. South American research has confirmed that pau d'arco has the ability to protect the liver, potentiate cancer therapies, shrink tumors and fight all kinds of infection.

The lapachol content of pau d'arco in combination with its other quinones gives it a significant antimicrobial and anti-tumor effect. It has successfully been used to treat yeast infections, vaginitis, tumors and blood disorders. Any ailment which may have blood toxicity at its root can be treated with pau d'arco. Conditions such as dermatitis, eczema, psoriasis, pernicious anemia, leukemia, allergies, asthma, etc. may respond to the blood purifying properties of pau d'arco. In addition, pau d'arco enhances immune function during any infection and protects the liver by boosting its ability to detoxify the blood. Concerning the viability of pau d'arco as a therapeutic and nutritive agent, Louise Tenney has written:

Pau d'arco is rich in calcium and iron, which are both essential for a healthy body and mind. Calcium is effective in helping to prevent disease and also protects the colon . . . iron is necessary for healthy blood. Selenium in this herb helps protect the immune system against diseases such as cancer. It [pau d'arco] also contains vitamin C, which is an antioxidant.[18]

Pau d'arco is said to contribute to the greater vitality of the body by boosting its organic defenses thereby revitalizing all body systems on a cellular level. It is believed to increase resistance to disease and promote a feeling a well being. Its ability to control pain has also been observed. It has been referred to as a powerful tonic and blood builder as well as an effective preventative and curative agent. Louise Tenney cites evidence of pau d'arco's stimulating effect on digestive and excretory systems, stating, "The Dietemann Research Foundation in Los Angeles, California found in extract samples that pau d'arco is stimulating to the alimentary tract through the rectum and then back to the liver, gallbladder and sweat gland."[19]

Consider the following quote from *Applied and Environmental Microbiology* concerning the properties of lapachol, one of the primary constituents of pau d'arco:

Lapachol is a naturally occurring naphthoquinone derivative found in the heartwood of several plants. It was first isolated and characterized during the late nineteenth century and the compound has been synthesized. Considerable attention has been focused on lapachol and its analogs, since these compounds possess antimalarial, antitumor, antibiotic and antischisotsosmal properties. Lapachol itself has been examined for its potential as an antitumor agent in phase I clinical trials.[20]

Dr. Daniel Mowrey also give evidence of pau d'arco's many therapeutic properties, stating:

Lapacho [pau d'arco] is applied externally and internally for the treatment of fevers, infections, colds, flu, syphilis, cancer, respiratory problems, skin ulcerations and boils, dysentery, gastrointestinal problems of all kinds, debilitating conditions such as arthritis and prostatitis and circulation disturbances. Other conditions reportedly cured with lapacho [pau d'arco] include lupus, diabetes, Hodgkin's diseases, osteomyelitis, Parkinson's disease and psoriasis. Lapacho [pau d'arco] is used to relieve pain, kill germs, increase the flow of urine, and even as an antidote to poisons. Its use in many ways parallels that of echinacea on this continent and ginseng in Asia, except that its actions appear to exceed them both in terms of its potential as a cancer treatment.[21]

As previously mentioned, ingesting lapachol as part of the whole pau d'arco bark is preferable to taking it as an isolated or synthesized drug. Ingesting pau d'arco in tea form by boiling lapacho tree bark provides a synergistic array of all of its quinones, which work together to create optimal therapeutic effects.

Pau d'arco tea also has the following less known actions: as an analgesic that diminishes pain without the loss of consciousness; as a sedative that helps to alleviate nervousness, irritation and distress; as a diuretic that stimulates secretion and flow of urine; and as a virucidal capable of inhibiting viral infections.[22]

THERAPEUTIC APPLICATIONS

Cancer

Interestingly, after word of the tumor-inhibiting attributes of pau d'arco reached this country, the National Cancer Institute initiated its own extensive studies of the lapachol compound. In 1968, lapachol was subjected to phase 1 clinical trials on the basis of tests which clearly demonstrated its antitumor capabilities. Consider the following quote:

> Some constituents or groups of constituents of lapacho have indeed been found to suppress tumor formation and reduce tumor viability, both in experimental animal trials and in clinical settings involving human patients. In addition, anecdotal data abound to such an extent that to overlook its importance is to turn one's back on a potentially invaluable source of aid and health.[23]

Clinical studies evaluating the use of pau d'arco for cancer in South America had already shown that it does have significant anti-cancer properties. Pau d'arco constituents seems to attack malignant cells. Extracts of pau d'arco bark were shown to inhibit the growth of animal tumors by 44 percent. Lapachol was found to inhibit various types of malignancies.[24] Using pau d'arco in combination with chemotherapy has been successful in some cases. An unexpected bonus of pau d'arco therapy was that it also has the ability to alleviate some kinds of pain normally associated with cancer.[25]

Currently, no official American medical opinion on the effectiveness of pau d'arco as a cancer treatment exists due to the fact that cancer testing was subsequently halted after 1970. Michael Murray, in his book, *The Healing Power of Herbs*, expresses his disappointment that typical medical approaches to herb testing. Regarding the NCI's decision to halt lapachol testing, he stated:

> The approach [reason for terminating lapachol tests] . . . indicates a flaw in the underlying philosophy of the pharmaceutical sciences and the NCI program. Since the initial studies involved the whole plant, the detailed studies should have been undertaken with the whole plant; some of the

other quinones have also been shown to have anticancer activities.[26]

Varro E. Tyler of Dean of the School of Pharmacy at Purdue University stated that lapachol clearly proved that it had significant activity against Walker 256 carcinoma, particularly when administered orally to animals implanted with this tumor. It was subsequently found to be active against Yoshida sarcoma, Murphy-Sturm sarcoma and to possess some antibiotic and antischistosomal activity.

Lapachol is very quickly absorbed through the walls of the gastrointestinal tract after ingesting it orally. Tissue uptake is seen except in brain and blood cells. Concerning tumor tissue, Michael Murray has stated that "a significant amount appears in the tumor after 6 hours, with most of the drug disappearing from the other body tissues."[27]

The way in which pau d'arco attacks tumors is based on its ability to uncouple the mitochondrial oxidative phosphorylation that only occurs in malignant cells.[28] The ability of pau d'arco to discriminate between healthy and cancerous cells and target only those that are diseased is what makes the herb so valuable. The ability of herbs to selectively treat diseased cells without harming healthy cells is what makes them such remarkable therapeutic agents. Pharmaceutical drugs, radiation, chemotherapy etc. do not have this selective ability. While this booklet in no way advocates abandoning standard cancer treatments, the potential value of pau d'arco in treating tumors should be investigated. *(Note:* Using pau d'arco to augment standard cancer treatments should be done under the care of a qualified physician.)

Leukemia

Dr. Daniel Mowrey has stated that "leukemia has proven particularly susceptible to the application of lapacho and several of its constituents. Some researchers feel the lapacho is one of the most important antitumor agents in the entire world."[29] The following quote provides one account of pau d'arco's affect on leukemia:

> Dr. Ruiz, as of 1968, successfully treated three cases of leukemia with extracts from pau d'arco. One case was that of five-year old Maria Adela Vera. On July 15, 1967, doctors at the Concepcion hospital has lost hope of saving her life. Her cytological table had been steadily worsening and indicated as imminent fatal issue . . . Maria Adela, after ingesting for six days teas and elixirs of pau d'arco, was much better . . . the improvement continued until the leucocytes were down to 6500 and the platelets had increased to 135,000 . . . the last analysis of her blood was made in the following September, 1967 and showed 4.2 million erythrocytes and 160,000 platelets. And so Maria Adela was discharged . . .[30]

Press reports also told of other cases of lymphatic leukemia that responded to pau d'arco tea treatment. Maria's recovery was reported in several Brazilian newspapers including *La Razon*, published in Buenos Aires on Nov. 6, 1967.

One study published in 1975 reported that lapachol demonstrated significant activity against lymphocytic leukemia in mice.[31] This particular form of lapachol was taken from *Tabebuia avellandedae*, or pau d'arco.

Notwithstanding the above information, many hundreds of anecdotal reports have emerged from South America dealing with the ability of pau d'arco to inhibit certain tumors or even cure some cases of cancer.

Antibacterial Properties

Initial testing conducted when lapachol was first isolated from the bark of the pau d'arco tree revealed that it possessed significant antibacterial activity. Tests proved that it inhibited both gram positive and acid-fast bacteria as well as the *Brucella* bacterial strain.[32] Apparently, this particular quinone kills certain microorganisms by inhibiting the metabolic processes which supply energy. Subsequent tests continued to suggest that substances from the bark demonstrated a specific antibiotic action against not only bacteria but fungi as well.[33] The subsequent discovery of at least 15 more quinones led to more research which found that several other of these compounds also showed strong antimicrobial and antifungacidal properties.

In time tests revealed that specific quinones were more effective against certain kinds of microorganisms. Xyloidone was effective against *Staphylococcus aureus, Candida albicans,* kurzei and neopfromans as well as the pathogens which cause tuberculosis, dysentery and anthrax.[35] Michael Murray, who has devoted an entire chapter of his book, *The Healing Power of Herbs,* to lapacho (pau d'arco), lists in table form all of the microorganisms which are affected by *Tabebuia avellandedae.* Referring to his table he writes:

> Several of the microorganisms listed are pathogenic, such as *Staphylococcus aureus* and the *Brucella* species. The causative agents of tuberculosis, dysentery, and anthrax are also inhibited by xyloidone. In addition to its activity against a variety of bacteria, this quinone inhibits several species of fungus including *Candida albicans, Candida kruzei* and *Candida neoformans.* Lapachol, like many naphthoquinones, acts as a respiratory poison by interfering with energy production in the microorganism.[36]

Can Pau d'Arco Kill Viruses?

Several of the chemical constituents of pau d'arco including lapachol have shown activity against several viruses including Herpes I and II, poliovirus, vesicular stomatitis virus and influenza.[37] The beta-lapachone quinone found in pau d'arco is considered a powerful anti-viral compound. Consider the following quote regarding its virus killing potential:

> In experiments with viruses, betalapachone demonstrated its ability to inhibit certain key viral enzymes, such as DNA and RNA polymerase, and retro virus reverse transcriptase. These actions have great significance in the possible treatment of acquired immuno deficiency syndrome (AIDS), Epstein-Barr virus and other viral infections.[38]

Terry Willard, Ph.D., also supports the existence of pau d'arco's antiviral properties, stating that "beta-lapachone inhibits Friend virus and Rous sarcoma virus in chickens."[39]

Yeast Infections

The astringent quality of pau d'arco in combination with its high naphthaquinone content make this herb an effective treatment against certain strains of *Candida* (yeast infections). It has been used with success against yeast infections that can frequently occur during or after antibiotic therapy and are unusually hard to control. Using extracts of pau d'arco on tampons to treat vaginal yeast infections has been successful in several cases.

Antiparasitic Action

A study published in the *American Journal of Tropical Medicine and Hygiene* addressed the ability of dietary lapachol to protect against *Schistosoma mansoni,* an infection caused by worms which penetrate the skin. The tests found that taking lapachol orally resulted in its secretion presumably by the sebaceous glands onto the skin where it acted as a surface barrier to worm penetration.[40] The fact that decaying lapacho trees do not become moldy or mildewed also supports the antifungal properties of its bark.

A Natural Anti-Inflammatory Agent

Extracts of pau d'arco have been used to treat both allergies and asthma which are triggered by environmental allergens. Dr. A. Volpini of San Paolo, Brazil has referred to the anti-inflammatory action of pau d'arco. He also considers it as an effective analgesic and sedative as well as an antiphlogistic (an agent which can subdue inflammation or fever). Michael Murray has stated that "extracts of the bark from *Tabebuia avellandedae* demonstrate clear anti-inflammatory activity with low toxicity."[41]

This particular property of pau d'arco combined with its analgesic effects strongly suggests that it may be a valuable treatment for joint diseases like arthritis. Taking daily doses of pau d'arco tea may be a great benefit for anyone with joint disease.

Analgesic Action

In studying the medicinal effects of pau d'arco, its pain relieving action subsequently emerged. When taken orally, the lapachol compound was found to produce significant reductions in pain associated with several forms of cancer, specifically liver, breast and prostate cancers. Its value for alleviating arthritic pain has also been observed.[42] The anti-inflammatory properties of this herb may account for its analgesic action.

Blood-builder and Tonic

Pau d'arco has also been shown to enhance blood function. Louise Tenney, M.H., states:

The writings from South America tell us that pau d'arco is a powerful tonic and blood builder which increases the hemoglobin content and number of red corpuscles. It gives the body greater vitality by strengthening its organic defenses. It seems to have the ability to revitalize the body by creating new vital elements and new normal cell growth. It increases bodily resistance and well-being. Pau d'Arco has neither contraindications nor incompatibilities. It permits the control of "incurable" illness, lengthening life without suffering . . . Pau d'arco acts as a blood tonic and helps the proper assimilation of nutrients and the elimination of wastes.[43]

An Overlooked Antioxidant

One of the little known attributes of pau d'arco is its ability to inhibit free radicals and other inflammatory agents on a cellular level. For this reason pau d'arco is considered by some to be an anti-aging herb. Today the intrinsic value of antioxidants as protective agents against degenerative diseases and aging processes has been wholeheartedly accepted in the scientific community. The fact that pau d'arco also encourages the production of red blood cells may help to boost its protective effect in facilitating better oxygenation of healthy tissue which promotes healing and disease prevention.

An Effective Laxative

Using pau d'arco for an extended period will help to ensure regularity of bowel movements. The quinones contained in the herb stimulate the bowel to evacuate much in the same way as cascara sagrada. The effect is gentle and usually does not create diarrhea or cramping.

Combining Pau d'Arco with other Medications

Considering how pau d'arco works with other agents, Louise Tenney tells us:

The articles from South America also state pau d'arco [taheebo] can be combined with other medications without fear, no matter how active the ingredients are. It helps to reduce counteraction to medications in general and especially to antibiotics, which allow other medications to work more effectively and helps reduce the danger of toxic effect upon the liver.[44]

Daniel B. Mowrey, Ph.D. in his book, *Herbal Tonic Therapies,* writes:

A common thread that runs throughout early and current empirical and clinical reports of lapacho [pau d'arco] treatment is the consistent observation that the herb eliminates many of the common side effects of the orthodox medications. There is no explanation of this action, but it is so often seen that on cannot easily doubt its validity. Pain, hair loss, and immune dysfunction are among the symptoms most commonly eliminated.[45]

HOW TO TAKE PAU D'ARCO

While dosages can vary according to need, pau d'arco tea or capsulized pau d'arco can be used several times a day over an extended period of time. If using dried bark products, the decoction should be boiled for at least 15 to 20 minutes. A cup of tea is taken from 2 to 8 times per day. Decoctions are usually made by boiling 1 teaspoon of pau d'arco for each cup of water for approximately 15 minutes.

In studying native uses of medicinal plants like pau d'arco, scientists have discovered that the herb in its whole form is well suited for continued use by mouth over long periods of time without the side effects of synthetic drugs. This particular attribute of whole botanicals seems particularly suited to meet the needs of primitive cultures. Unfortunately, commercial pharmaceutical interests have often overlooked the value of the whole plant in attempting to isolate its therapeutic components and mass produce its chemical compounds. (*Note:* Apparently studies have found that the lapachol constituent of pau d'arco is more effective when taken orally rather than through injections.) Mowrey believes this finding has important implications, stating:

> These results contradict a substantial amount of research on orthodox drugs that indicates the superiority of injectable routes. What is the meaning of this anomaly? Could it be a sign that the natural routes of administration (i.e, oral) are better suited for natural substances? The further removed from the natural state, the more active substances become when injected directly into the bloodstream and the less able the natural process of the body are in dealing with them.[46]

Environmental Concerns

Dr. Theodore Meyer, who is credited with bringing the therapeutic properties of pau d'arco to the attention of the medical establishment, was considered one of the leading South American botanists of this century. Among his many accomplishments, his ongoing effort to save the lapacho tree from destruction is one of his most admirable. His practice of hand stripping lapacho bark in Argentina resulted in leaving a majority of the bark untouched, thereby ensuring the life of the tree. For several decades now, Argentina has protected the country's lapacho trees under its "Save the Tree" program.

Herbs that Augment Pau d'Arco

- *For hypoglycemia:* licorice
- *For viral or bacterial infections:* garlic, echinacea, goldenseal
- *For fungal infections:* black walnut
- *For kidneys:* Alfalfa, marshmallow, burdock, kelp and yarrow
- *For the liver:* milk thistle
- *For blood purification:* red clover, dandelion, Oregon grape root

Primary Applications of Pau d'Arco

- AIDS
- blood disorders
- *Candida albicans*
- eczema
- Hodgkin's disease
- infections
- liver disease
- pain (especially arthritic)
- anemia
- cancer
- diabetes
- herpes
- hypoglycemia
- leukemia
- lupus
- parasites

- prostate disorders
- ringworm
- ulcers
- warts
- pyorrhea
- tumors
- venereal disease
- yeast infections

Secondary Applications of Pau d'Arco

- allergies
- boils
- colitis
- fever
- nephritis
- psoriasis
- asthma
- bronchitis
- dysentery
- gastritis
- Parkinson's disease
- skin ailments

SUMMARY OF PAU D'ARCO'S THERAPEUTIC APPLICATIONS

- Pau d'arco fights fungal and viral infections such as yeast and herpes while boosting immune function.
- Pau d'arco reduces tumors in some cases of cancer including leukemia.
- Pau d'arco has reduced the need for insulin in some insulin-dependent diabetics.
- Pau d'arco helps to eliminate the pain of arthritis and cancer as a natural anodyne.
- Pau d'arco facilitates the removal of toxins from the blood.
- Pau d'arco helps to strengthen the liver and remove poisons from liver tissue.
- Pau d'arco is good for any blood-born illness.
- Pau d'arco's high iron content boosts the assimilation of other nutrients.

Pau d'Arco

- Pau d'arco is thought to help fade age spots.
- Pau d'arco has anti-mutagenic properties.
- Pau d'arco works as a natural antibiotic, antiviral, antibacterial and antifungal agent.
- Pau d'arco inhibits free radicals and in this way is an anti-aging herb.
- Pau d'arco promotes gentle regularity.

ENDNOTES

1 Terry Willard, Ph.D., THE WILD ROSE SCIENTIFIC HERBAL. (Wild Rose College of Natural Healing, Calgary, Alberta: 1991), 198.

2 "Structure-Antitumor Activity Relationships among Quinone Derivatives," CANCER CHEMOTHERAPY REPORTS, Part 2, Vol. 4 No. 2, April, 1974.

3 "Early Clinical Studies with lapachol," CANCER CHEMOTHERAPY REPORTS, Part 2, Vol. 4, No. 4, December, 1974. See also L. F. Feiser, et al., "Naphthoquinone antimalarials, General Survey," JOURNAL OF THE AMERICAN CHEMICAL SOCIETY 70: 3156, 1948 and J. L. Howland, "Uncoupling and inhibition of oxidative phosphorylation by 2-hydroxy-3alkyl-1, 4-naphthoquinones," BIOCHEM. BIOPHYS. ACTA. 77:659, 1963.

4 Ara De Marderosian, Ph.D., and Lawrence E. Liberti M.S., NATURAL PRODUCT MEDICINE: A SCIENTIFIC GUIDE TO FOOD, DRUGS AND COSMETICS, (George Stickly Co., Philadelphia: 1988), 364.

5 A.R. Burnett and R.H. Thompson, "Naturally occurring quinones. X. The quinonoid constituents of Tabebuia avellandedae (Bignoniaceae), JOURNAL CHEM. SOC. (C), 2100-2104, 1967.

6 Michael T, Murray, N.D., THE HEALING POWER OF HERBS (Prima Publishing, Rocklin, California: 1992), 221. See also R.K. Morrison, et al., "Oral toxicology studies with lapachol," TOXICOL. APPL. PHARMACOL. 17: 1-11, 1970.

7 Ibid., 226.

8 Daniel B. Mowrey, Ph.D., HERBAL TONIC THERAPIES. (Keats Publishing, New Canaan, Connecticut: 1993), 83.

9 Murray, 226.

10 Ibid., 221.

11 Ibid.

12 Mowrey, 72.

13 Ibid. See also S.C. Hooker, "Constitution of lapachol and its derivatives. The structure of the anylene chain." JOURNAL CHEM. SOCIETY, 89: 1356, 1896.

14 Murray 222. See also Burnett and Thompson.

15 Bob Borino, "1,000-year old Inca Cancer Cure Works," GLOBE, vol. 28, no. 37, Sept. 15, 1981.

16 Murray, 224.

17 J.B. Block, et al., "Early clinical studies with lapachol," (NSC-11905), CANCER CHEMOTHERAPY REPORT, 4: 27-28, 1974.

18 Louise Tenney, M.H., THE ENCYCLOPEDIA OF NATURAL REMEDIES. (Woodland Publishing, Pleasant Grove, Utah: 1995), 80.

19 Louise Tenney, M.H., "Pau d'Arco (Tabebuia altissima)." TODAY'S HERBS, vol. III, no. 9, 2-3, May, 1983.

20 Sharee Otten and John P. Rosazza, "Microbial Transformations of Natural Antitumor agents: oxidation of lapachol by Penicillium notatum," APPLIED AND ENVIRONMENTAL MICROBIOLOGY, vol. 35, no. 3, 554-57, March 1978.

21 Mowrey, 71.

22 Tenney, "Pau d'Arco, "2-3.

23 Mowrey, 75.

24 Marderosian 364. See also K.V. Rao, et al., CANCER RESEARCH, 28: 1952, 1968.

25 Jack Ritchason, THE LITTLE HERB ENCYCLOPEDIA, (Woodland Publishing, Pleasant Grove, Utah: 1994), 168. See also Mowrey, 77.

26 Murray, 224.

27 Ibid., 225.

28 Mowrey, 81.

29 Ibid., 75.

30 Carlos Hugo Burgstaller, "La Vuelta a los Vegetales," Buenos Aires, 1968.

31 M. Da Consolacae, F. Linardi, et al., "A lapachol Derivative Active against Mouse Lymphocytic Leukemia," SECTION OF PHARMACOLOGY, Instituto Biologico, Sao Paolo, Brazil, March 13, 1975, 388.

32 Murray 222.

33 Ibid.

34 Ibid. See also H. Gershon and L. Shanks "Fungitoxicity of 1,4-naphtho-quinones to Candida albicans and Truchophyton mentagrophytes," CAN. J. MICROBIOLOGY. 21, 1317-21, 1975.

35 Ibid.

36 Ibid.

37 Ibid.

38 Ibid.

39 Willard, 200. See also K Schaffner-Sabba, et al., "b lapachone: synthesis of derivatives and activities in tumour models," JOURNAL OF MEDICINAL CHEMISTRY. 27: 990-994, 1984.

40 Frederick G. Austin, "Schistosoma Mansoni Chemoprophylaxis with Dietary lapachol," THE AMERICAN JOURNAL OF TROPICAL MEDICINE AND HYGIENE. Vol. 23, no. 3, 1974: 412.

41 Murray, 225.

42 Mowrey, 77.

43 Tenney, "Pau d'Arco," 2.

44 Ibid., 3.

45 Mowrey, 73.

46 Ibid., 76.